Table of Contents

INTRODUCTION

The testicles and ovaries produce testosterone. Producing too little or too much testosterone can affect your physical and mental health. Testosterone is a hormone found in humans, as well as in other animals. In men, the testicles primarily make testosterone. Women's ovaries also make testosterone, though in much smaller amounts.The production of testosterone starts to increase significantly during puberty and begins to dip after age 30 or so.

Testosterone is most often associated with sex drive and plays a vital role in sperm production. It also affects bone and muscle mass, the way men store fat in the body, and even red blood cell production. A man's testosterone levels can also affect his mood.

Low testosterone levels

Low levels of testosterone, also called low T levels, can produce a variety of symptoms in men, including:

decreased sex drive

less energy

weight gain

feelings of depression

moodiness

low self-esteem

less body hair

thinner bones

While testosterone production naturally tapers off as a man ages, other factors can cause hormone levels to drop. Injury to the testicles and cancer treatments such as chemotherapy or radiation can negatively affect testosterone production.

Chronic health conditions and stress can also reduce testosterone production. Some of these include:

AIDS

kidney disease

alcoholism

cirrhosis of the liver

Testosterone levels decline steadily in adult women, however, low T levels can also produce a variety of symptoms, including:

low libido

reduced bone strength

poor concentration

depression

Low T levels in women can be caused by removal of the ovaries as well as diseases of the pituitary, hypothalamus, or adrenal glands. Testosterone therapy may be prescribed for women with low T levels, however, the treatment's effectiveness on improving sexual function or cognitive function among postmenopausal women is unclear.

Testing testosterone

A simple blood test can determine testosterone levels. There's a wide range of normal or healthy levels of testosterone circulating in the bloodstream. Normal male testosterone levels range between 280 and 1,100 nanograms per deciliter (ng/dL) for adult males, and between 15 and 70 ng/dL for adult females, according to the University of Rochester Medical Center. Ranges can vary among different labs, so it's important to speak with your doctor about your results.

If an adult male's testosterone levels are below 300 ng/dL, a doctor may do a workup to determine the cause of low testosterone, according to the American Urological Association. Low testosterone levels could be a sign of pituitary gland problems. The pituitary gland sends a signaling hormone to the testicles to produce more testosterone. A low T test result in an adult man could mean the pituitary gland isn't working properly. But a young teen with low testosterone levels might be experiencing delayed puberty.

Moderately elevated testosterone levels in men may produce few noticeable symptoms. Boys with higher levels of testosterone may begin puberty earlier. Women with high testosterone may develop masculine features. Abnormally high levels of testosterone could be the result of an adrenal gland disorder, or even cancer of the testes.. High testosterone levels may also occur in less serious conditions. For example, congenital adrenal hyperplasia, which can affect males and females, is a rare but natural cause for elevated testosterone production. If your testosterone levels are extremely high, your doctor may order other tests to find out the cause.

Testosterone replacement therapy
Reduced testosterone production, a condition known as hypogonadism, doesn't always require treatment. You may be a candidate for testosterone replacement therapy if low T is interfering with your health and quality of life.

Artificial testosterone can be administered orally, through injections, or with gels or skin patches. Replacement therapy may produce desired results, such as greater muscle mass and a stronger sex drive. But the treatment does carry some side effects. These include:

oily skin

fluid retention

testicles shrinking

decrease in sperm production

Some studies have found no greater risk of prostate cancer with testosterone replacement therapy, but it continues to be a topic of ongoing research. One study suggests that there's a lower risk of aggressive prostate cancers for those on testosterone replacement therapy, but more research is needed.

Testosterone is most commonly associated with sex drive in men. It also affects mental health, bone and muscle mass, fat storage, and red blood cell production. Abnormally low or high levels can affect a man's mental and physical health. Your doctor can check your testosterone levels with a simple blood test. Testosterone therapy is available to treat men with low levels of testosterone. If you have low T, ask your doctor if this type of therapy might benefit you.

LOW TESTOSTERONE IN MEN

Low testosterone levels can affect your libido and cause physical changes, sleep issues, and trouble with emotional regulation. Treatment can increase testosterone levels or treat symptoms. Testosterone is a hormone found in humans. Men have much higher levels of testosterone than women. Production increases during puberty and starts to decrease after age 30. For each year over age 30, the level of testosterone in men starts to slowly dip at a rate of around 1 percent per year. A decrease in testosterone level is a natural result of aging. Testosterone helps maintain a number of important bodily functions in men, including:

sex drive

sperm production

muscle mass/strength

fat distribution

bone density

red blood cell production

Because testosterone affects so many functions, its decrease can bring about significant physical and emotional changes.

Sexual function

Testosterone is the hormone most responsible for sex drives and high libidos in men. A decrease in testosterone can mean a decrease in libido. One of the biggest worries faced by men with declining testosterone levels is the chance that their sexual desire and performance will be affected. As men age, they can experience a number of symptoms related to sexual function that may be a result of lowered levels of this hormone. These include:

reduced desire for sex

fewer erections that happen spontaneously, such as during sleep

infertility

Erectile dysfunction (ED) is not commonly caused by low testosterone production. In cases where ED accompanies lower testosterone production, hormone replacement therapy may help your ED. These side effects typically don't happen suddenly. If they do, lower testosterone levels may not be the only cause.

Physical changes

A number of physical changes can happen to your body if you have low testosterone levels. Testosterone is sometimes referred to as the "male" hormone. It helps increase muscle mass, leads to body hair, and contributes to an overall masculine form. Decreases in testosterone can lead to physical changes including the following:

increased body fat

decreased strength/mass of muscles

fragile bones

decreased body hair

swelling/tenderness in the breast tissue

hot flashes

increased fatigue

effects on cholesterol metabolism

Sleep disturbances

Low testosterone can cause lower energy levels, insomnia and other changes in your sleep patterns. Testosterone replacement therapy may contribute to or cause sleep apnea. Sleep apnea is a serious medical condition that causes your breathing to stop and start repeatedly while you sleep. It can disrupt your sleep pattern in the process and raise your risk for other complications, like having a stroke. On the other hand, changes in the body that occur as a result of sleep apnea can lead to low testosterone levels. Even if you don't have sleep apnea, low testosterone can still contribute to a decrease in the hours of sleep. Researchers aren't yet sure why this happens.

Emotional changes

In addition to causing physical changes, having low levels of testosterone can affect you on an emotional level. The condition can lead to feelings of sadness or depression. Some people have trouble with memory and concentration and experience lowered motivation and self-confidence. Testosterone is a hormone that affects emotional regulation.

Depression has been linked to men with low testosterone. This could result from a combination of the irritability, decreased sex drive, and fatigue that can come with low testosterone.

Other causes
While each of the symptoms above may be a result of a lowered testosterone level, they may also be normal side effects of aging. Other reasons that you might experience some of these symptoms include:

a thyroid condition

injury to testicles

testicular cancer

infection

HIV

type 2 diabetes

side effects of medications

alcohol use

genetic abnormalities that affect the testicles

pituitary gland problems

To determine what's causing these symptoms for you, schedule an appointment with your doctor.

Treatment

Regardless of the reason you're experiencing low testosterone, treatment options are available to increase testosterone or reduce unwanted side effects.

Testosterone therapy

Testosterone therapy can be delivered in several ways:

injections into the muscle every few weeks

patches or gels applied to the skin

a patch that is applied inside the mouth

pellets that are inserted under the skin of the buttocks

Testosterone therapy is not recommended for those who have experienced or are at a high risk of prostate cancer.

Losing weight and being physically active

Exercising more and losing weight can help slow the decrease of testosterone your body is experiencing.

Erectile dysfunction medication

If your most concerning symptom from lower testosterone is erectile dysfunction, erectile dysfunction medications may help.

Sleeping aids

If you're unable to get relief from insomnia using relaxation and natural remedies, sleeping medications may help.

If you're experiencing any symptoms of low testosterone, ask your doctor to test your levels. A diagnosis can be made with a simple blood test, and there are a variety of treatment options to reduce unwanted side effects of low T. Your doctor can also help you determine if there's an underlying cause triggering your low testosterone.

High Testosterone Levels in Women

Certain health conditions may cause high testosterone in females. You may experience symptoms like balding or acne.

Women with high testosterone

Testosterone is a male sex hormone, or androgen, produced in a woman's ovaries in small amounts. Combined with estrogen, the female sex hormone, testosterone helps with the growth, maintenance, and repair of a woman's reproductive tissues, bone mass, and human behaviors.

Age (in years) Testosterone range (in nanograms per deciliter)

10–11 < 7–44

12–16 < 7–75

17–18 20–75

19+ 8–60

The range for males is higher, depending on age:

Age (in years) Testosterone range (in nanograms per deciliter)

10–11 < 7–130

12–13 < 7–800

14   < 7–1,200

15–16 100–1,200

17–18 300–1,200

19+   240–950

An imbalance of testosterone in the female body can have damaging effects on a woman's health and sex drive.

Symptoms of too much testosterone in women
Too much testosterone can cause symptoms that affect a woman's physical appearance including:

excess body hair, specifically facial hair

balding

acne

enlarged clitoris

decreased breast size

deepening of the voice

increased muscle mass

Overly high levels of testosterone in women can also cause:

irregular menstrual cycles

low libido

changes in mood

In more severe cases of testosterone imbalances in women, high testosterone can cause infertility and obesity.

Diagnosing high testosterone
If you notice any of the symptoms listed above, you should talk to your doctor. Your doctor will perform a physical examination based on your symptoms to determine whether or not you need additional tests. During the examination, your doctor will look for these symptoms:

abnormal facial hair

acne

excess body hair

If your symptoms seem to be abnormal, your doctor will suggest a testosterone test to measure hormone levels in your blood. To perform this test, your doctor will draw some of your blood and have it examined for hormone levels. The test is typically performed in the morning when testosterone levels are at their highest. Prior to performing this test, your doctor may ask you to stop taking any prescriptions that could affect the test results.

Causes of high testosterone in women
Various diseases or hormonal disorders can cause hormonal changes in women. The most common causes of high testosterone levels in women are hirsutism, polycystic ovary syndrome, and congenital adrenal hyperplasia.

1. Hirsutism

Hirsutism is a hormonal condition in women that causes growth of unwanted hair, specifically on the back, face, and chest. The amount of body hair growth is highly dependent on genetics, but this condition is primarily caused by an imbalance of androgen hormones.

2. Polycystic ovary syndrome

Polycystic ovary syndrome (PCOS) is another hormonal disorder caused by an excess of androgen hormones in women. If you have PCOS, you may have irregular or prolonged periods, unwanted body hair growth, and enlarged ovaries that may not function properly. Other common complications of PCOS are:

infertility

miscarriage

type 2 diabetes

obesity

endometrial cancer

3. Congenital adrenal hyperplasia

Congenital adrenal hyperplasia (CAH) is a disorder that directly affects the adrenal glands and the production of the body's hormones. In many cases of CAH, the body overproduces androgen. Common symptoms of this disorder in women include:

infertility

masculine characteristics

early appearance of pubic hair

severe acne

Treatment options

Treatment for high testosterone depends on the cause, but generally includes medication or lifestyle changes. Medications used to treat high testosterone include:

glucocorticosteroids

metformin

oral contraceptives

spironolactone

Oral contraceptives have been shown as effective treatment for blocking testosterone, but this treatment method will interfere if you have immediate plans to get pregnant. According to research from the American Academy of Family Physicians, low-dose birth control that use low levels of norgestimate, gestodene, and desogestrel are the best choices. All of these medications are only available by prescription. To obtain one, you must meet with your doctor or gynecologist.bMaking certain lifestyle changes can also affect testosterone levels. Starting an exercise or weight loss program can help because losing weight can improve symptoms. Some women choose only to treat their symptoms, including shaving or bleaching hair and using facial cleaners for acne or oily skin.

If you're experiencing symptoms of high testosterone levels, meet with your doctor. They will be able to find the cause and come up with a treatment plan specific to you.

WHAT'S CAUSING MY LOW TESTOSTERONE?

Low testosterone (low T), also called male hypogonadism, may be caused by many things, such as aging, hormone changes, chemotherapy, and others. Treatment involves taking various forms of testosterone. Low testosterone (low T) affects 4 to 5 million men in the US. Testosterone is an important hormone in the human body. But it starts to decrease each year after age 30Trusted Source. In some men this can be substantial. Between 19 and 39 percent of older menTrusted Source may have low levels of testosterone.

Older men with low T have increasingly sought testosterone replacement therapy (TRT) in recent years. TRT addresses symptoms such as low libido, poor muscle mass, and low energy. It's not just older men that are affected by low T. Young men, even babies and children, can also have this problem.

Symptoms of low T

Low levels of testosterone that are atypical of normal aging are due to other primary or secondary causes of hypogonadism. Hypogonadism in males happens when the testicles don't produce enough testosterone. Hypogonadism can start during fetal development, during puberty, or during adulthood.

Fetal development

If hypogonadism begins during fetal development, the primary result is impaired growth of external sex organs. Depending on when hypogonadism starts and the level of testosterone present during fetal development, a male child can develop:

female genitals

ambiguous genitals, neither clearly male or female

underdeveloped male genitals

Puberty

Normal growth can be jeopardized if hypogonadism occurs during puberty. Problems occur with:

muscle development

deepening of the voice

lack of body hair

underdeveloped genitals

overly long limbs

enlarged breasts (gynecomastia)

Adulthood

Later in life, insufficient testosterone can lead to other problems. Symptoms include:

low energy levels

low muscle mass

infertility

erectile dysfunction

decreased sex drive

slow hair growth or hair loss

loss of bone mass

gynecomastia

Fatigue and mental fogginess are some commonly reported mental and emotional symptoms in men with low T.

Causes of low testosterone

The two basic types of hypogonadism are primary and secondary hypogonadism.

Primary hypogonadism

Underactive testes cause primary hypogonadism. That's because they don't manufacture sufficient levels of testosterone for optimal growth and health. This underactivity can be caused by an inherited trait. It can also be acquired by accident or illness. Inherited conditions include:

Undescended testicles: When the testicles fail to descend from the abdomen before birth

Klinefelter's syndrome: A condition in which a man is born with three sex chromosomes: X, X, and Y.

Hemochromatosis: Too much iron in the blood causes testicular failure or pituitary damage

Types of testicle damage that can lead to primary hypogonadism include:

Physical injury to the testicles: Injury must occur to both testicles to affect testosterone levels.

Mumps orchitis: A mumps infection can injure testicles.

Cancer treatment: Chemotherapy or radiation can damage testicles.

Secondary hypogonadism

Secondary hypogonadism is caused by damage to the pituitary gland or hypothalamus. These parts of the brain control hormone production by the testes. Inherited or disease conditions in this category include:

Pituitary disorders caused by drugs, kidney failure, or small tumors

Kallmann syndrome, a condition connected to abnormal hypothalamus function

Inflammatory diseases, such as tuberculosis, sarcoidosis, and histiocytosis, which can impact the pituitary gland and the hypothalamus

HIV/AIDS, which can affect the pituitary gland, hypothalamus, and testes

Acquired circumstances that can lead to secondary hypogonadism include:

Normal aging: Aging affects production and response to hormones.

Obesity: High body fat can affect hormone production and response.

Medications: Opioid pain meds and steroids can affect function of the pituitary gland and hypothalamus.

Concurrent illness: Severe emotional stress or physical stress from an illness or surgery can cause the reproductive system to temporarily shut down.

You may be affected by primary, secondary, or a mixed hypogonadism. Mixed hypogonadism is more common with increased age. People undergoing glucocorticoid therapy can develop the condition. It also can affect people with sickle-cell disease, thalassemia, or alcoholism.

Changes you can make

If you're experiencing symptoms of low T, lifestyle changes may help to ease your symptoms. A good first step is increasing activity levels and maintaining a healthy diet in order to reduce body fat. It can also be helpful to avoid glucocorticoid medications such as prednisone as well as opioid pain medications.

Testosterone replacement

If lifestyle changes don't work for you, you may need to begin testosterone replacement therapy (TRT) for treatment of low T. TRT can be very important for helping teenage males with hypogonadism experience normal masculine development. Sufficient testosterone levels help maintain health and well-being in adult males.

Q: How long does it take for testosterone injections to start working?

Anonymous

A: Testosterone, when given intramuscularly, is slowly absorbed. It's therefore administered at intervals of 2–4 weeks. Levels peak 2–3 days after an injection and slowly decline until the next dose is given.

Everyone is different, so some people will see improvement in symptoms within a few weeks, while others will need more time to notice any changes. This is mostly dependent on factors such as age and underlying medical conditions. On average, it takes about 3 weeks to see an improvement in sexual desire (libido), energy, and mood. Changes in erections are slower and may take up to 6 months.

Testosterone replacement also affects metabolic parameters with effects on cholesterol occurring in 4 weeks, peaking at

6–12 months and blood sugar levels improving after 3–12 months. Other changes take much longer. You can expect a change in muscle strength and body composition (fat mass/lean body mass) within 12–16 weeks. Effects on bone mineral density are seen after 6 months with the full effect occurring around 2 years.

How to Manage Low Testosterone and Your Sex Life

Low testosterone causes more than just problems with sex drive. It can also affect your mood, sleep, and energy levels, which can disrupt your quality of life and relationships. If you want to keep your relationship healthy, a good start is to learn more about how low testosterone affects your body and how to communicate with your partner about your symptoms.

The effects of low testosterone

Testosterone helps support a number of bodily functions in men, including sex drive (libido), muscle strength, bone density, and sperm production. Symptoms of low testosterone (low T) may start gradually as testosterone levels fall below normal.

Reduced sexual function

Testosterone is the key hormone responsible for a man's sex drive. With low T, you might notice a considerable reduction in the desire for sex. You might also have fewer spontaneous erections during sleep. In some cases, you might still desire sex but be unable to maintain an erection. This is known as erectile dysfunction.

Mood changes

When men with low T visit their doctors, they often report unhappiness, fatigue, irritability, lack of focus, or trouble sleeping. Though testosterone is linked to emotional regulation, it's still unclear whether these mood changes are a direct cause of low T or a byproduct of some of its symptoms, like sexual performance issues or poor sleep. "I believe it is a mistake to only focus on any one factor, be it the biological or just the psychological or just the interpersonal," Dr. Daniel B. Singley, a board certified psychologist and President-Elect of the APA Society for the Psychological Study of Men & Masculinities, told Healthline.

"I think it's really critical to take a biopsychosocial approach because when you drill into the experience of folks who have testosterone that's elevated or low or depression and/or sexual dysfunction, what you see is they all go together, and they impact each other in fairly nuanced and sometimes kind of unexpected ways." Men often worry how their sexual performance will be affected by low T. They may even feel a sense of shame when they're unable to perform. In a 2015 studyTrusted Source, for example, men seeking treatment for borderline testosterone had a significantly higher rate of depression compared to the general population. A lack of energy and feelings of inadequacy and shame can be confusing for both people in a relationship.

How to talk with your partner

Sexual dysfunction can bring about feelings of embarrassment or shame, but it's important not to withdraw and avoid telling your partner what's going on. "People need to communicate and communicate proactively and fully, including not just 'the what,' but the 'what it means to me,'" explained Singley. In other words, it's important to go further than just saying you're having trouble with your libido. Explain to your partner what's hard about it, what your insecurities are, and that you've already been assessed by a doctor.t

It's also important not to play the blame game. When dealing with such sensitive topics, Singley explains, it's helpful to talk about the facts and your own personal experience rather than shutting down or blaming your partner. That said, your partner may blame themselves and wonder if they're simply not attractive to you. "They're essentially sort of making it about themselves, oftentimes in a subliminal or sort of subconscious way that most of us do to kind of pretend that we have a sense of control over something that, in fact, we don't," explained Singley. It's a good idea to emphasize that it's not their fault. And it's not yours, either.

While you have the right to talk about this, Singley says, the conversation will likely go better if you lead with "honest curiosity and grace."

Managing low testosterone

Testosterone levels decrease naturally as men age: About 40% of men over the age of 45 have low testosterone. But medications and lifestyle changes can help improve symptoms.

Medication
Your doctor can prescribe testosterone replacement therapy (TRT), which is available as injections, patches, gels, and implantable pellets. TRT may increase your risk of cardiovascular disease, but more research is needed about its long-term safety. Before starting treatment, talk with your doctor about the risks and benefits.nIt's important to note that TRT shouldn't be used when testosterone levels are considered normal. Increasing levels can have serious adverse effects. It can also cause the body to stop naturally producing testosterone.

Lifestyle changes

You may be able to increase your testosterone levels naturally by:

exercising

managing stress

avoiding excess alcohol

improving sleep quality

maintaining a moderate weight

Therapy

Counseling or talk therapy can help treat the psychological symptoms of low T and help you navigate relationship concerns that arise from it. It's hard to talk about sex, and even couples who have been together for a while may still need to work on their communication.

Low testosterone is usually treatable, but you'll need to be proactive in getting the help you need. It can feel embarrassing to bring up issues with sexual function with a doctor or partner. Education and open communication can go a long way in improving your symptoms.

Many men may feel self-conscious about discussing sexual issues with a doctor, but doing so can greatly improve your health and your relationship. Once diagnosed with low testosterone, communicating with your partner can help relieve stress as you wait for treatment to work. If you're having trouble coping or communicating about the effects of low testosterone, sex therapy or counseling can help bridge that gap.

LOW SEX DRIVE: COMMON CAUSES AND TREATMENT

It's natural to sometimes lose interest in sex, but long-term low libido may have an underlying cause. It may stem from low testosterone, lack of sleep, depression or stress, substance use, and more. If changes in your sex drive concern you, a physician can offer more guidance. Low libido describes a decreased interest in sexual activity.

It's common to lose interest in sex from time to time, and libido levels vary through life. It's also normal for your interest not to match your partner's at times. However, low libido for a long period of time may cause concern for some people. It can sometimes be an indicator of an underlying health condition. Here are a few potential causes of low libido in men.

Low testosterone

Testosterone is an important male hormone. In men, it's mostly produced in the testicle. Testosterone is responsible for building muscles and bone mass, and for stimulating sperm production. Your testosterone levels also factor into your sex drive. Normal testosterone levels will vary. However, adult men are considered to have low testosterone, or low T, when their levels fall below 300 nanograms per deciliter (ng/dL), according to guidelines from the American Urological Association (AUA). When your testosterone levels decrease, your desire for sex also decreases. Decreasing testosterone is a normal part of aging. However, a drastic drop in testosterone can lead to decreased libido. Talk to your doctor if you think this might be an issue for you. You may be able to take supplements or gels to increase your testosterone levels.

Medications

Taking certain medications can lower testosterone levels, which in turn may lead to low libido. For example, blood pressure medications such as ACE inhibitors and beta-blockers may prevent ejaculation and erections. Other medications that can lower testosterone levels include:

chemotherapy or radiation treatments for cancer

hormones used to treat prostate cancer

corticosteroids

opioid pain relievers, such as morphine (MorphaBond, MS Contin) and oxycodone (OxyContin, Percocet)

an antifungal medication called ketoconazole

cimetidine (Tagamet), which is used for heartburn and gastroesophageal reflux disease (GERD)

anabolic steroids, which may be used by athletes to increase muscle mass

certain antidepressants

If you're experiencing the effects of low testosterone, talk to your doctor. They may advise you to switch medications.

Restless legs syndrome (RLS)

Restless legs syndrome (RLS) is the uncontrollable urge to move your legs. A study found that men with RLS are at higher risk for developing erectile dysfunction (ED) than those without RLS. ED occurs when a man can't have or maintain an erections. In the study, researchers discovered that men who had RLS occurrences at least five times per month were about 50 percent more likely to develop ED than men without RLS. Also, men who had RLS episodes more frequently were even more likely to become impotent.

Depression

Depression changes all parts of a person's life. People with depression experience a reduced or complete lack of interest in activities they once found pleasurable, including sex. Low libido is also a side effect of some antidepressants, including:

serotonin-norepinephrine reuptake inhibitors (SNRIs), such as duloxetine (Cymbalta)

selective serotonin reuptake inhibitors (SSRIs), like fluoxetine (Prozac) and sertraline (Zoloft)

However, the norepinephrine and dopamine reuptake inhibitor (NRDI) bupropion (Wellbutrin SR, Wellbutrin XL) hasn't been shown to reduce the libido.

Talk to your doctor if you're taking antidepressants and you have a low libido. They might address your side effects by adjusting your dose or having you switch to another medication.

Chronic illness

When you're not feeling well due to the effects of a chronic health condition, such as chronic pain, sex is likely low on your list of priorities. Certain illnesses, such as cancer, can reduce your sperm production counts as well. Other chronic illnesses that can take a toll on your libido include:

type 2 diabetes

obesity

high blood pressure

high cholesterol

chronic lung, heart, kidney, and liver failure

If you're experiencing a chronic illness, talk with your partner about ways to be intimate during this time. You may also consider seeing a marriage counselor or sex therapist about your issues.

Sleep problems

A study in the Journal of Clinical Sleep Medicine found that nonobese men with obstructive sleep apnea (OSA) experience lower testosterone levels. In turn, this leads to decreased sexual activity and libido. In the study, researchers found that nearly one-third of the men who had severe sleep apnea also had reduced levels of testosterone. In another recent studyTrusted Source in young, healthy men, testosterone levels were decreased by 10 to 15 percent after a week of sleep restriction to five hours per night. The researchers found that the effects of restricting sleep on testosterone levels were especially evident between 2:00 pm and 10:00 pm the next day.

Aging

Testosterone levels, which are linked to libido, are at their highest when men are in their late teens. In your older years, it may take longer to have orgasms, ejaculate, and become aroused. Your erections may not be as hard, and it may take longer for your penis to become erect. However, medications are available that can help treat these issues.

Stress

If you're distracted by situations or periods of high pressure, sexual desire may decrease. This is because stress can disrupt your hormone levels. Your arteries can narrow in times of stress. This narrowing restricts blood flow and potentially causes ED. One study published in Scientific Research and Essays supported the notion that stress has a direct effect on sexual problems in both men and women.

Another studyTrusted Source of veterans with post-traumatic stress disorder (PTSD) found that the stress disorder increased their risk of sexual dysfunction more than threefold.. Stress is hard to avoid. Relationship problems, divorce, facing the death of a loved one, financial worries, a new baby, or a busy work environment are just some of the life events that can greatly affect the desire for sex.

Stress management techniques, such as breathing exercises, meditation, and talking to a therapist, may help. In one study, for example, men who were newly diagnosed with ED showed significant improvement in erectile function scores after participating in an 8-week stress management program.

Low self-esteem

Self-esteem is defined as the general opinion a person has about their own self. Low self-esteem, low confidence, and poor body image can take a toll on your emotional health and well-being. If you feel that you're unattractive, or undesirable, it'll likely put a damper on sexual encounters. Not liking what you see in the mirror can even make you want to avoid having sex altogether. Low self-esteem may also cause anxiety about sexual performance, which can lead to issues with ED and reduced sexual desire. Over time, self-esteem issues can result in larger mental health problems, such as depression, anxiety, and drug or alcohol abuse — all of which have been linked to low libido.

Too little (or too much) exercise

Too little or too much exercise can also be responsible for low sex drive in men. Too little exercise (or none at all) can lead to a range of health problems that can affect sexual desire and arousal. Getting regular exercise may reduce your risk for chronic conditions such as obesity, high blood pressure, and type 2 diabetes, all of which are associated with low libido. Moderate exercise is known to lower cortisol levels at night and reduce stress, which can help increase sex drive. On the other hand, over-exercising has also been shown to affect sexual health. In one study, higher levels of chronic intense and lengthy endurance training on a regular basis were strongly associated with decreased libido scores in men.

Alcohol

Heavy alcohol drinking, or more than 14 mixed drinks in a week, has also been linked to a decrease in testosterone production. Over a long period of time, excessive amounts of alcohol can reduce your sex drive. The Cleveland Clinic recommends that men who consume more than three or more alcoholic beverages regularly should consider drinking less. The Centers for Disease Control and PreventionTrusted Source suggest that an average adult male should have two or fewer alcoholic beverages daily; any more than this can lead to long-term health deterioration.

Drug use

In addition to alcohol, the use of tobacco, marijuana, and illicit drugs such as opiates has also been connected to a decrease in testosterone production. This can result in a lack of sexual desire. Smoking has also been found to have a negative impact on sperm production and sperm movement.

Physical and emotional side effects of low libido

A decreased sex drive can be very unsettling for men. Low libido can lead to a vicious cycle of physical and emotional side effects, including ED — the inability to maintain an erection long enough to have satisfactory sex. ED may cause a man to experience anxiety around sex. This can lead to tension and conflicts between him and his partner, which may in turn lead to fewer sexual encounters and more relationship issues. Failure to perform due to ED can trigger feelings of depression, self-esteem issues, and poor body image.

Treating low libido often depends on treating the underlying issue.If low libido is caused by an underlying health condition, you may need to switch medications. If your low libido has psychological causes, you may need to visit a therapist for relationship counseling. You can also take steps to boost your libido on your own. The following actions have the potential to increase your libido:

living a healthier lifestyle

getting enough sleep

practicing stress management

eating a healthier diet

Could Low Testosterone Be Causing Your Brain Fog?

Testosterone's primary functions are sexual desire and function. However, low testosterone may also impact cognition, leading to symptoms like brain fog. Researchers are finding that testosterone affects more than just your sex life. The hormone may play a part in brain health, cognition, and the way you think. Keep reading to learn more about the connections between testosterone, brain fog, and thinking.

How does testosterone affect your brain?

Testosterone is a type of hormone called androgen. There are specific androgenTrusted Source receptors within the brain. Think of these receptors as light switches that only androgen hormones can activate. The hormone can also cross the blood-brain barrier. This barrier is a protective mechanism in your brain designed to keep out substances that could potentially damage it, and allow other substances like medications in. The fact that testosterone can cross the blood-brain barrier means that it could affect your thinking or brain functioning. Testosterone may also have protective effects on the brain, including:

delaying nerve cell death

improving nerve cell regrowth after damage

reducing the effects of nerve damage

having anti-inflammatory actions on the nerves

These are just some of the potentially protective benefits to the brain that researchers think testosterone may have. We're sure to learn more in the coming years as studies continue.

Language matters

In this article, we use "male and female" to refer to someone's sex as determined by their chromosomes, and "men and women" when referring to their gender, unless quoting from sources using nonspecific language. The studies cited within the article frequently do not delineate between sex and gender and can be assumed to have entirely cisgender participants. Sex is determined by chromosomes, and gender is a social construct that can vary between time periods and cultures. Both of these aspects are acknowledged to exist on a spectrum both historically and by modern scientific consensus.

Can low testosterone cause brain fog or other mental problems?
Cognitive decline tends to occur with aging. Testosterone levels tend to decrease with aging as well. Some smaller studies suggest that men with lower testosterone levels tend to have poorer cognitive function than men the same age with higher testosterone levels. Sometimes, low testosterone levels can cause symptoms like difficulty maintaining an erection or low sex drive. These are the symptoms people typically connect with low testosterone. However, it may also cause other symptoms, such as:

affected memory

fatigue or low energy levels

reduced physical strength

increased irritability

higher instances of depression

If you have these symptoms and can't identify another underlying cause like staying up late at night or eating a poor diet, low testosterone levels could play a role. Most of the studies that connect testosterone with improving mental function are on older males. This is because they may be more impacted by changes in memory function. That said, a 2021 study found that higher testosterone levels may reduce the ability to perform thinking tasks in younger males.

What happens if low testosterone goes untreated?
Low testosterone can cause symptoms like low sex drive, reduced lean muscle mass, and erectile dysfunction. You may also have difficulty focusing and lower energy levels, yet not know these symptoms are related to low testosterone. Although low testosterone may affect your overall health and well-being, it doesn't typically lead to

life threatening conditions. An exception is that low testosterone can cause weakened bones, which increases your risk for osteoporosis.

How do you fix low testosterone?

Doctors can prescribe different forms of testosterone to help increase low levels, including:

injections

intranasal

oral/buccal dose

testosterone gel

testosterone pellets embedded under the skin

topical patches

Speak with a healthcare professional before taking any testosterone supplements because they may have side effects. For example, gel testosterone can be troublesome if you have young children.

Will testosterone help with brain fog?

Although some smaller studies and individual case reportsTrusted Source suggest that taking testosterone may help improve brain fog, a bigger meta-analysis suggests there's no proven benefit. As such, there's no consensus to fully support that taking testosterone creates changes in thinking or memory.

What hormones cause brain fog?

Hormonal changes due to menopause, pregnancy, stress, and other factors may lead to brain fog. Some hormones may include:

testosterone

androgen

estrogen

progesterone

cortisol

What are the effects of high testosterone on the brain?

In their summary of current research, the authors of a 2021 study suggest that high levels of testosterone in the brain may affect the recognition of social cues and emotions in children and young adults.

Low testosterone can affect your energy levels and thinking, which could contribute to brain fog. Unfortunately, researchers haven't yet established whether testosterone replacement therapy can alter these effects. More research is needed to support that testosterone supplements may be beneficial for your brain fog. If you think you may have low testosterone levels, talk with a doctor about testing and potential treatments.

ALL ABOUT THE MALE SEX DRIVE

There are many stereotypes that portray men as sex-obsessed machines. Books, television shows, and movies often feature characters and plot points that assume men are crazy about sex and women are only concerned with romance.

Stereotypes about male sex drive

So what stereotypes about the male sex drive are true? How do men compare to women? Let's look at these popular myths about male sexuality.

Men think about sex all day long

A recent study at Ohio State University of over 200 students debunks the popular myth that men think about sex every seven seconds. That would mean 8,000 thoughts in 16 waking hours! The young men in the study reported thoughts of sex 19 times per day on average. The young women in the study reported an average of 10 thoughts about sex per day. So do men think about sex twice as much as women? Well, the study also suggested that men thought about food and sleep more frequently than women. It's possible that men are more comfortable thinking about sex and reporting their thoughts. Terri Fisher, the lead author of the study, claims that people who reported being comfortable with sex in the study's questionnaire were most likely to think about sex on a frequent basis.

Men masturbate more often than women

In a study conducted in 2009 on 600 adults in Guangzhou, China, 48.8 percent of females and 68.7 percent of males reported that they had masturbated. The survey also suggested that a significant number of adults had a negative attitude toward masturbation, particularly women.

Men usually take 2 to 7 minutes to orgasm

Masters and Johnson, two important sex researchers, suggest a Four-Phase Model for understanding the sexual response cycle:

excitement

plateau

orgasm

resolution

Masters and Johnson assert that males and female both experience these phases during sexual activity. But the duration of each phase differs widely from person to person. Determining how long it takes a man or a woman to orgasm is difficult because the excitement phase and the plateau phase may begin several minutes or several hours before a person climaxes.

Men are less romantic than women

As suggested by Masters and Johnson's Four-Phase Model, sexual excitement is different for everyone. Sources of arousal can vary greatly from person to person. Sexual norms and taboos often shape the way that men and women experience sexuality and can impact the way they report it in surveys. This makes it difficult to scientifically prove that men are biologically not inclined toward romantic arousal.

Sex drive and the brain

Sex drive is usually described as libido. There is no numeric measurement for libido. Instead, sex drive is understood in relevant terms. For example, a low libido means a decreased interest or desire in sex. The male libido lives in two areas of the brain: the cerebral cortex and the limbic system. These parts of the brain are vital to a man's sex drive and performance. They are so important, in fact, that a man can have an orgasm simply by thinking or dreaming about a sexual experience.

The cerebral cortex is the gray matter that makes up the outer layer of the brain. It's the part of your brain that's responsible for higher functions like planning and thinking. This includes thinking about sex. When you become aroused, signals that originate in the cerebral cortex can interact with other parts of the brain and nerves. Some of these nerves speed up your heart rate and blood flow to your genitals. They also signal the process that creates an rection. The limbic system includes multiple parts of the brain: the hippocampus, hypothalamus and amygdala, and others. These parts are involved with emotion, motivation, and sex drive. Researchers at Emory UniversityTrusted Source found that viewing sexually arousing images increased activity in the amygdalae of men more than it did for women. However, there are many parts of the brain involved with sexual response, so this finding does not necessarily mean that men are more easily aroused than women.

TESTOSTERONE

Testosterone is the hormone most closely associated with male sex drive. Produced mainly in the testicles, testosterone has a crucial role in a number of body functions, including:

development of male sex organs

growth of body hair

bone mass and muscle development

deepening of the voice in puberty

sperm production

production of red blood cells

Low levels of testosterone are often tied to a low libido. Testosterone levels tend to be higher in the morning and lower at night. In a man's lifetime, his testosterone levels are at their highest in his late teens, after which they slowly begin to decline.

Loss of libido

Sex drive can decrease with age. But sometimes a loss of libido is tied to an underlying condition. The following can cause a decrease in sex drive:

Stress or depression. If you are experiencing mental health issues, talk to your doctor. He or she may prescribe medication or suggest psychotherapy.

Endocrine disorders. An endocrine disorder may decrease male sex hormones.

Low testosterone levels. Certain medical conditions, like sleep apnea, can cause low testosterone levels, which can impact your sex drive.

Certain medications. Some medications can impact your libido. For instance, some antidepressants, antihistamines, and even blood pressure medications can impair erections. Your doctor may be able to suggest an alternative.

High blood pressure. Damage to the vascular system can hurt a man's ability to get or maintain an erection.

Diabetes. Like having high blood pressure, diabetes can damage a man's vascular system and affect his ability to maintain an rection. Only you can measure what is normal for your sex drive. If you are experiencing libido changes, talk to your doctor. Sometimes it can be difficult to talk to someone about your sexual desires, but a medical professional may be able to help you.

Does the male sex drive ever go away? For many men, the libido will never completely disappear. For most men, libido will certainly change over time. The way you make love and enjoy sex will likely change over time as well, as will the frequency. But sex and intimacy can be a pleasurable part of aging.

10 Ways to Boost Male Fertility and Increase Sperm Count

Staying active, minimizing stress, and making changes to your diet and lifestyle can help support male fertility. Certain supplements may also be beneficial for increasing sperm count. If you and your partner are experiencing fertility issues, know that you're not alone. Infertility is more common than you might think. It affects about one in every six couples, and researchers estimate about one in every three cases is due to fertility problems in the male partner alone. While infertility is not always treatable, there are some things you can do to boost your chances of conceiving. Fertility can sometimes be improved with a healthy diet, supplements, and other lifestyle strategies.

What is male infertility?

Fertility refers to people's ability to reproduce without medical assistance. Male infertility is when a man has a poor chance of making his female partner pregnant. It usually depends on the quality of his sperm cells. Sometimes infertility is linked to sexual function, and other times it could be linked to semen quality. Here are some examples of each:

Libido. Otherwise known as sex drive, libido describes a person's desire to have sex. Foods or supplements that claim to increase libido are called aphrodisiacs.

Erectile dysfunction. Also known as impotence, erectile dysfunction is when a man is unable to develop or maintain an erection.

Sperm count. An important aspect of semen quality is the number or concentration of sperm cells in a given amount of semen.

Sperm motility. An essential function of healthy sperm cells is their ability to swim. Sperm motility is measured as the percentage of moving sperm cells in a sample of semen.

Testosterone levels. Low levels of testosterone, the male sex hormone, may be responsible for infertility in some men.

Infertility can have multiple causes and may depend on genetics, general health, fitness, diseases, and dietary contaminants.

Additionally, a healthy lifestyle and diet are important. Some foods and nutrients are associated with greater fertility benefits than others. Here are 10 science-backed ways to boost sperm count and increase fertility in men.

1. Take D-aspartic acid supplements

D-aspartic acid (D-AA) is a form of aspartic acid, a type of amino acid that's sold as a dietary supplement. It should not be confused with L-aspartic acid, which makes up the structure of many proteins and is far more common than D-AA. D-AA is mainly present in certain glands, such as the testicles, as well as in semen and sperm cells. Researchers believe that D-AA is implicated in male fertility. In fact, D-AA levels are significantly lower in infertile men than fertile men. This is supported by studies showing that D-AA supplements may increase levels of testosterone, the male sex hormone that plays an essential role in male fertility.

For example, a study in infertile men suggested that taking 2.7 grams of D-AA for 3 months increased their testosterone levels by 30–60% and sperm count and motility by 60–100%. The number of pregnancies also increased among their partners (4). Another controlled study in healthy men showed that taking 3 grams of D-AA supplements daily for 2 weeks increased testosterone levels by 42% (5Trusted Source).

However, the evidence is not consistent. Studies in athletes or strength-trained men with normal to high testosterone levels found that D-AA didn't increase its levels further and even reduced them at high doses. The current evidence indicates that D-AA supplements may improve fertility in men with low testosterone levels, while they don't consistently provide additional benefits in men with normal to high levels. More research is needed to investigate the potential long-term risks and benefits of D-AA supplements in humans.

2. Exercise regularly

Besides being good for your general health, exercising regularly can boost testosterone levels and improve fertility. Studies show that men who exercise regularly have higher testosterone levels and better semen quality than inactive men. However, you should avoid too much exercise, as it may have the opposite effect and potentially reduce testosterone levels. Getting the right amount of zinc can minimize this risk. If you rarely exercise but want to improve your fertility, make becoming physically active one of your top priorities.

3. Get enough vitamin C

You're probably familiar with vitamin C's ability to boost the immune system. Some evidence indicates that taking antioxidant supplements, such as vitamin C, may improve fertility. Oxidative stress is when levels of reactive oxygen species (ROS) reach harmful levels in the body. It happens when the body's own antioxidant defenses are overwhelmed because of disease, old age, an unhealthy lifestyle, or environmental pollutants. ROS are constantly being produced in the body, but their levels are kept in check in healthy people. High levels of ROS may promote tissue injury and inflammation, increasing the risk of chronic disease. There's also some evidence that oxidative stress and excessively high levels of ROS may lead to infertility in men. Taking in enough antioxidants, such as vitamin C, may help counteract some of these harmful effects. There's also some evidence that vitamin C supplements may improve semen quality.

A study in infertile men showed that taking 1,000-mg vitamin C supplements twice a day for up to 2 months increased sperm motility by 92% and sperm count by more than 100%. It also reduced the proportion of deformed sperm cells by 55%. Another observational study in Indian industrial workers suggested that taking 1,000 mg of vitamin C five times a week for 3 months may protect against DNA damage caused by ROS in sperm cells. Vitamin C supplements also significantly improved sperm count and motility, while reducing the numbers of deformed sperm cells. Taken together, these findings suggest that vitamin C may help improve fertility in infertile men with oxidative stress. However, controlled studies are needed before any definite claims can be made.

4. Relax and minimize stress

It's hard to get in the mood when you're feeling stressed, but there might be more to it than not feeling up for sex. Stress may reduce your sexual satisfaction and impair your fertility. Researchers believe the hormone cortisol may partly explain these adverse effects of stress. Prolonged stress raises levels of cortisol, which has strong negative effects on testosterone. When cortisol goes up, testosterone levels tend to go down. While severe, unexplained anxiety is typically treated with medication, milder forms of stress can be reduced with relaxation techniques. Stress management can be as simple as taking a walk in nature, meditating, exercising, or spending time with friends.

5. Get enough vitamin D

Vitamin D can be important for male and female fertility. It's another nutrient that may boost testosterone levels. One observational study showed that vitamin-D-deficient men were more likely to have low testosterone levels. A controlled study in 65 men with low testosterone levels and vitamin D deficiency supported these findings. Taking 3,000 IU of vitamin D3 every day for 1 year increased their testosterone levels by around 25%. High vitamin D levels are linked to greater sperm motility, but the evidence is inconsistent.

6. Try tribulus terrestris

Tribulus terrestris, also known as puncture vine, is a medicinal herb frequently used to enhance male fertility. One study in men with low sperm counts showed that taking 6 grams of tribulus root twice daily for 2 months improved erectile function and libido.

While Tribulus terrestris does not raise testosterone levels, research indicates that it may enhance the libido-promoting effects of testosterone. However, further studies are needed to confirm its aphrodisiac properties and evaluate the long-term risks and benefits of supplementing with it.

7. Take fenugreek supplements

Fenugreek (Trigonella foenum-graecum) is a popular culinary and medicinal herb. One study in 30 men who strength-trained four times a week analyzed the effects of taking 500 mg of fenugreek extract daily. The men experienced significantly increased testosterone levels, strength, and fat loss, compared with a placebo. Another study in 60 healthy men showed that taking 600 mg of Testofen, a supplement made from fenugreek seed extract and minerals, daily for 6 weeks improved libido, sexual performance, and strength (36Trusted Source).

These findings were confirmed by another, larger study in 120 healthy men. Taking 600 mg of Testofen every day for 3 months improved self-reported erectile function and the frequency of sexual activity. Also, the supplement significantly increased testosterone levels. Keep in mind that all of these studies examined fenugreek extracts. It's unlikely that whole fenugreek, which is used in cooking and herbal tea, is as effective.

8. Get enough zinc

Zinc is an essential mineral found in high amounts in animal foods, such as meat, fish, eggs, and shellfish. Getting enough zinc is one of the cornerstones of male fertility. Observational studies show that low zinc status or deficiency is associated with low testosterone levels, poor sperm quality, and an increased risk of male infertility. Also, taking zinc supplements increases testosterone levels and sperm count in those who are low in zinc.

Furthermore, zinc supplements may reduce the decreased testosterone levels that are associated with excessive amounts of high-intensity exercise. Controlled trials need to confirm these observational findings.

9. Consider ashwagandha

Ashwagandha (Withania somnifera) is a medicinal herb that's been used in India since ancient times. Studies suggest that ashwagandha may improve male fertility by boosting testosterone levels. One study in men with low sperm cell counts showed that taking 675 mg of ashwagandha root extract per day for 3 months significantly improved fertility. Specifically, it increased sperm counts by 167%, semen volume by 53%, and sperm motility by 57%, compared with levels at the start of the study. In comparison, minimal improvements were detected among those who got a placebo treatment. Increased testosterone levels may be partly responsible for these benefits.

A study in 57 young men following a strength-training program showed that consuming 600 mg of ashwagandha root extract daily significantly increased testosterone levels, muscle mass, and strength, compared with a placebo. These findings are supported by observational evidence indicating that ashwagandha supplements may improve sperm counts, sperm motility, antioxidant status, and testosterone levels (44Trusted Source, 45Trusted Source).

10. Eat maca root

Taking maca root supplements may improve libido, as well as fertility and sexual performance. Maca root is a popular plant food that originated in central Peru. Traditionally, it has been used for its ability to enhance libido and fertility. Several studies in men showed that taking 1.5–3 grams of dried maca root for periods of up to 3 months improved self-reported sexual desire or libido. Studies also suggest that maca root may improve sexual performance. In men with mild erectile dysfunction, taking 2.4 grams of dried maca root for 12 weeks slightly improved self-reported erectile function and sexual well-being. Taking 1.75 grams of maca root powder every day for 3 months also increased sperm count and motility in healthy men.

These findings have been partly confirmed by reviews, but the researchers noted that the evidence is weak and more research is needed before definite claims can be made. Additionally, maca root doesn't seem to affect hormone levels. Taking 1.5–3 grams of maca root per day for 3 months had no effects on testosterone or other reproductive hormones in healthy, fertile men.

CONCLUSION

Many things can help boost fertility, but what works for you depends on the cause of your fertility issues. Also, keep in mind that fertility and libido usually go hand in hand with your general health. For this reason, anything that improves your overall health is likely to boost your fertility.